The Home Workout Handbook

D1727707

Raza Imam

Get More Free Tips

My wife is a registered dietitian and I'm a fitness nut. Check out my blog for some great fitness tips. Here are my top articles:

- 37 Mind-Blowing Tips to Burn Fat & Build Muscle (w/ pics and links)
- How to Burn Fat & Get Ripped Eating One Meal per Day
- The 39 Coolest Fitness Blogs in the World (plus their most mind-blowing articles)
- The AMAZING Health Benefits of Greek Yogurt for Weight Loss and Bodybuilding
- 6 "Dirty" Secrets the Fitness Industry Uses to Make Billions (don't fall for these tricks)

Please share these articles on Facebook and Twitter!

And while you're there, don't forget to sign up to my email newsletter where I share free tips, updates, and exclusive articles.

I'll even give you a copy of my free report
"The ULTIMATE Muscle-Building Dessert"
https://goo.gl/sQjbsz

Get access to all of this at my blog:

www.TheScienceofGettingRipped.com

Notice

No part of this report may be reproduced or transmitted in any form whatsoever, electronic, or mechanical, including photocopying, recording, or by any informational storage or retrieval system without including the name of the author.

Disclaimer and Legal Notices

The information provided in this book is for educational purposes only. I am not a doctor and this is not meant to be taken as medical advice. The information provided in this book is based upon my experiences as well as my interpretations of the current research available. The advice and tips given in this course are meant for healthy adults only. You should consult your physician to insure the tips given in this course are appropriate for your individual circumstances. If you have any health issues or pre-existing conditions, please consult with your physician before implementing any of the information provided in this course. This product is for informational purposes only and the author does not accept any responsibilities for any liabilities or damages, real or perceived, resulting from the use of this information.

Can I Ask You a Quick Favor?

If you like this book, I would greatly appreciate if you could leave an honest review on Amazon.

Reviews are very important to us authors, and it only takes a minute to post. At the end of this book please post a review.

Also, please check out my comprehensive manual, *"The Science of Getting Ripped"* for workout plans and tips to burn fat and build muscle.

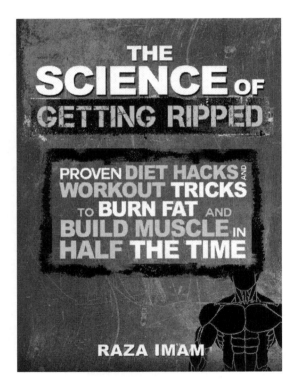

Click here to check it out

http://a.co/f0xlu1F

Thank you in advance!

Table of Contents

Who This Is For

This is for the average guy who wants to lose fat and build muscle. It's for the busy parent, the entrepreneur, the guy who wants to help others. He needs the physical strength to accomplish his goals, but also the discipline, fortitude, mental toughness, character, and self-respect to handle life's most difficult tasks.

Whether that means turning around a struggling business, volunteering with young kids, or raising a growing family, having a solid physique in addition to the inner strength to blast through life's obstacles and challenges is the key to success.

The ideal reader doesn't want to be a pretty boy fitness model nor a bodybuilder. He reads popular men's health magazines, is interested in technology, and photography, and current events, and sports. He is tech savvy and forward thinking, with aspirations and ambitions for himself and his family. He doesn't want to spend hours a day in the gym. He looks for efficiency and fitness hacks to get him the most results from his workouts.

Here's the thing, most products focus on getting ripped, and this will show you how to do just that. But the way I see it, you don't walk around with your shirt off all day. You DO meet people, solve problems, create plans, help others, encounter obstacles, and live a full life. So why not focus on not only the physical benefits you'll get when you workout, but on the confidence and mental toughness you gain as well? Seems like the best of both worlds to me.

My Story

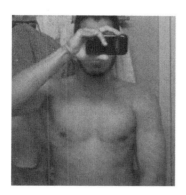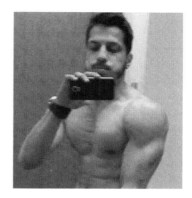

Like most 30-something guys with kids, I have a very busy life. Here's my typical day: An hour-long commute to and from work. Helping my 5 year-old with homework. Giving the kids baths. Putting them to bed. Doing dishes. Hanging out with the wife. And going to bed.

I love working out and used to be heavily involved in martial arts. But I just couldn't keep it up with this crazy schedule. I've been wanting to get back in shape for quite a while, but never had the time to go to the gym consistently. Once I hit 30, I was terrified that I would get the dreaded "skinny fat" body type. You know what I'm talking about. Skinny body with a pot belly.

Now I'm 34 with 3 kids and decided to start writing to help other people get in shape.

Sincerely,

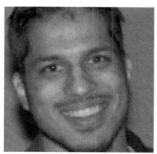

Raza Imam

Start With the End in Mind: Create a Goal and Visualize Yourself Achieving It

One of the best self-help books of all time is Psycho-Cybernetics written by Dr. Maxwell Maltz in the 1960's. He was a plastic surgeon that noticed patients who have had their limbs amputated still felt pain that limb.

Even though it had been amputated.

This got him thinking about self-image. He concluded that we become what we think about. He's not the first one to say this, but it really resonated with me.

The whole point of his book is that your mind is like a "heat seeking missile" If it has a goal, infused with emotion and passion, it will figure out how to accomplish it.

There will be trial and error, but if you keep believing in your goal and take action, you will eventually achieve it. He gives the example of a baby reaching for an object on a table. When he first reaches for it, he might miss, but he will eventually get it.

So belief creates a positive self-image. When you create a positive self-image of yourself ALREADY having accomplished your goal, you will have the motivation and drive to figure out it.

So here's a sample daily reminder that I set for myself on my phone. It pops up every morning at 6:30am. I read it every day to help me accomplish my goals:

"I have dropped body fat and am gradually building lean muscle now because I do reverse pyramid training twice a week. I got it by doing one heavy lift and two assistance lifts everytime I hit the gym. I do heavy reps for my main lift of 4-6 reps. I do 3 sets of 10

reps on my assistance lifts. I make sure that I lift explosively and take 3 seconds to lower the weight.

I also do 3 HIIT sessions per week which consist of 10 burpees, 10 jump lunges, 10 mountain climbers, and 10 high knees. I rest for one minute and repeat 4 more times.

I keep a 24 ounce water bottle at work and drink it 3 times before lunch. I then drink one after lunch to hit 100 ounces of water per day.

I keep greek yogurt, chocolate almonds, blueberries, and whey protein powder at work. I will eat 2 cups of greek yogurt with chocolate almonds and blueberries, along with 2 scoops of vanilla whey to hit 100 grams of protein. This helps me kill my sugar cravings. Eating like this makes diet adherence MUCH easier. Less prep time and less money.

I eat simple meals at home: grilled chicken, rice, boiled sweet potatoes, and grilled vegetables. I cook once or twice a week and keep this in the fridge to make meal planning easy."

I read this everyday and it lays out my ENTIRE plan to get ripped. Strength training. Diet. Cardio. Motivation. Everything.

Feel free to use it yourself.

Why I Love Working Out at Home (and why it's so good for you)

Working out in a gym is awesome.

The biggest reason I like working out in a gym is the equipment (duh!)

Squats, bench presses, overhead presses, deadlifts, bars to do weighted dip and pullups, and a range of dumbbells.

Everyone knows how effective these exercises are at building muscle and strength.

But for the longest time, I didn't.

I used to practice martial arts in high school and after college and always had the (wrong) impression that lifting weights is not good for you because it makes you "bulky", slow, and stiff.

Well, as I started reading more, I realized that I was <u>dead</u> wrong.

In fact, eating too much makes you bulky. And not stretching on your off days makes you inflexible.

Anyone who thinks that weight lifting makes you slow and bulky obviously knows nothing about explosive movements like power cleans, and high pulls, and jerks, and snatches.

At least I didn't.

Olympic sprinters (who are some of the leanest, most muscular athletes on the planet) do these weight lifting exercises and are not big, or bulky, or slow by any means.

Personally, I think some people in the fitness world have to bash others in order to justify their own positions. I feel that's what some martial arts guys would do to weightlifters.

Anway, the more I learned, the more I realized how wrong I was about weights.

So began my love affair with lifting.

I used many routines, starting with dumbbell circuit training. I would do a set of dumbbell presses, followed by a set of dumbbell rows, followed by a set of dumbbell squats. Then I'd rest for 90 seconds and do it all over again.

It allowed me to get stronger AND it had build in cardio because I was doing 3 sets of exercises in a row and wasn't resting very long until I did the same circuit all over again.

It was good, but then I started reading about barbell training.

Eventually, I learned about the StrongLifts 5x5 workout and decided to try it out. I instantly fell in love with squats, and deadlifts, and bench presses, and overhead presses.

But as I progressed, and the weight got heavier, it took me longer and longer to do my workouts.

And because I have a gym at work, I started spending upwards of an hour and a half in the gym during my lunch break.

I couldn't sustain that without raising eyebrows in the office. People were wondering why I was gone so long.

Then I switched to Starting Strength, which is similar to StrongLifts 5x5, except Mark Rippetoe recommends a few other exercises (power clean instead of rows) and recommends 3 sets of 5 reps as opposed to 5 sets of 5 reps.

Starting Strength was great, except that I never really learned how to do the power clean correctly (we didn't have bumper plates at the gym at my job)

After a few months, my younger brother, who is a 6'4" 285lb powerlifter, told me about Jim Wendler's 5/3/1 program.

When I read about it I really liked it. It focused on one or two main lifts per day, with 2-3 accessory lifts.

It's a very smart way to train after you graduate from Starting Strength because it focuses on making very small changes over time; either in the amount of reps you do, or the amount of weight that you lift.

So I continued with that program for a while and enjoyed it a lot.

Then I read about Reverse Pyramid Training (RPT) and it made the most sense to me.

With RPT, you warm up and then do your heaviest set first, and then for your next sets you use lighter weights but did more reps.

Out of all of the workout styles I experimented with, RPT was my absolute favorite because it was efficient, fast, and got me results (I was stronger and leaner than I had ever been).

During this time I developed a bit of elitism. Maybe because I read too many Mark Rippetoe articles where he constantly praised barbells. Maybe because I viewed myself as tougher and stronger than I actually was. Maybe because I *wanted* to feel superior.

Whatever the case, I would see guys do dumbbell workouts in the gym, or bodyweight workouts, and I would ever so slightly look down on them. Not in an arrogant or mean way, but it a *"if only you knew how much better barbells are"* kind of way.

The sad thing is that my wife actually wanted to work out with me at home. And because I was in love with lifting barbells in the gym, I missed an opportunity to workout at home with her.

I was focused on getting bigger and stronger in the big lifts (squat, bench press, overhead press, and deadlift) and didn't want to stop progressing.

Now there's nothing wrong with that, but if your wife is literally asking you to work out with her, you can't let fitness dogma get in the way of spending time with your family.

I was so stupid…

All the while, I was accumulating little injuries here and there from squatting or deadlifting or overhead pressing too much weight. Nothing that seriously incapacitated me, but it was enough to cause a noticeable amount of pain.

Well, things were going good, until I overhead pressed 135 pounds (I weight 160lbs at the time) and felt a sharp pain on the lower right side of my back. That little injury caused me to scale the weight back on my overhead press quite a bit.

Dang, I thought… I was actually making good progress and now I had to go back.

Well, I still kept working out, but I made sure I used weights that I could actually handle.

I also paid **extreme** attention to my form so that I didn't hurt myself.

One more thing I did was focus on the proper workout tempo. In other words, I read about how lifting weights explosively makes you stronger and burns more fat, and how lowering the weight slowly does the same (I cover this topic in detail later in this book)

So like I said, things were going good. I was injury free again, going to the gym 3 times a week, getting stronger.

But then I found out that my wife was having a baby (our third).

And at that point I knew, once the baby is born, I won't be able to workout in the gym as much.

So I had to come up with a different plan.

I didn't want to forgo working out in the gym, so I started to workout in the gym twice a week and at home twice a week.

And it was a GREAT program. It was one that I created myself and it suited my goals perfectly.

Well, once our baby was born, I didn't go to the gym for 4 months. I was so sleep deprived from waking up in the middle of the night that I didn't want to go in the gym, lift heavy weights, and injure myself because I couldn't recover properly (you get stronger when you rest, so sleep is **crucial**)

The good news is that by this time, I'd grown past my "*barbells are superior*" phase and realized that as long as I'm lifting the proper amount of weights at the right tempo, it doesn't matter what I use; barbells, dumbbells, bodyweight exercises, kettlebells, etc.

Also, as my young family grows, they need me more. Like I mentioned earlier, I have a 2 hour daily commute, when I get home my kids need to eat dinner with me, and spend time playing with me, and need help with their homework, and my wife needs a break.

I can't selfishly take another hour and a half out of the day to go to the gym.

It's funny how things come full circle. At first I was dogmatic about bodyweight exercises because I thought weights make you "*slow and bulky*". Then I got into weights because I thought that people who exclusively do bodyweight exercises are destined to be weak and small. And now I'm praising bodyweight exercises again.

The point is to be safe and consistent – not tied to dogma.

Because blindly following dogma leads to injuries, and can have you miss out on the benefits of bodyweight exercises.

Afterall, guys who strictly train with heavy barbells now regret it.

Mark Rippetoe has had multiple injuries in his weight lifting career.

My younger brother (the powerlifter I mentioned earlier) broke his foot and bulged a disc in his back from doing inhuman lifts (700lb squat, 650lb deadlift, 315lb overhead press!)

Guys like Jim Wendler and Jason Ferruggia and Elliott Hulse and Omar Isuf (all guys that I admire and respect) have had horrible, horrible injuries from punishing their bodies so much.

As these guys get older (and as I get older), they realize the importance of keeping their muscles, joints, and tendons healthy – not just getting bigger and stronger and more "jacked".

And that's the thing, if these weight lifting pro's all realize that they need to be more careful with their bodies, then I need to do the same thing.

The funny thing is that all of these guys will agree with me and say that pushups are incredible for healing your shoulders, and how planks help with hip pain, and how back bridges and glute ham raises are good for your back and hips.

The lesson is not to blindly criticize – not even CrossFit (some fitness people love it, and others love to hate it)

Afterall, I'm not a powerlifter or a competitive bodybuilder. I'm a 30 something IT guy with a wife and 3 beautiful kids that depend on me. I don't need to be the next Arnold Schwarzeneggar or Dwayne Johnson.

These guys' entire lifestyles revolve around working out and lifting weights. They can afford to take the time to recooperate (or at least take steroids that help them recover faster).

But I can't.

And you know what the worst thing is with doing heavy barbell lifts?

It's that if you get sick for a week, or get injured, or can't keep working out because you're travelling, or working more, or having a baby, or some other major life event occurs – you lose your progress.

My younger brother told me about a fellow powerlifter that squatted 1000lbs (yes, 1000 pounds!)

Well, the guy got the flu and couldn't lift weights for a week. When he got back in the gym, he was only able to squat 800lbs ("only" 800 pounds, LOL)

The point is that he lost 200 pounds of strength just from being out of the gym for a week.

I have another friend that weight 160lbs and could bench 320lbs. But he stopped going to the gym for a few months because he got a new job, and now he can barely bench press 205lbs.

And that's why, despite how much I love lifting heavy barbells in the gym, I'm returning back to home workouts that rely on my own bodyweight, dumbbells, kettlebells, and plyometrics.

So I'm going to show you how to burn fat, build muscle, build explosive strength, and get ripped with home workouts that you can do consistently, and that are arguably safer and faster than doing big barbell movements in a gym.

I'll get off of my soapbox now.

I just wanted to say that bodyweight exercises are great. Barbell exercises are great. Kettlebells and dumbbells are great. They're all great.

And in this book I want to share my years of experience with you so that you can get the best results while working out at home.

What You'll Need

Now, if you want to workout at home, you're going to need a few basic things. I'm going to list everything you could possibly buy for an ultimate home gym. But to be clear, not all of these items are required, in fact just a few of them are. Either way, I'll tell you the benefits of each one and whether or not they're required or not.

- **Pull-up Bar**: A pullup bar is not absolutely essential if you can't do a pullup or a chinup. But if you can, then it's required. Pullups and chin-ups are great for building your forearms, back, and biceps. The variety of grips and positions you can use activate those muscles from various angles. Most pullup bars cost less than $30 from stores like Target, Walmart, etc. You can also get cheaper ones from Amazon, Ebay or Craigslist.

- **Gymnastic Rings**: Gymnastic rings are becoming incredibly popular these days. Strength coach Jason Ferruggia has said that rings are the greatest tool for building upper body strength. They allow you to do all sorts of pull-ups, chin-ups, dips, inverted rows, and even pushups. So if you can easily perform those movements, you'll want to invest in a quality set of rings so they last you a lifetime. If you're advanced, you'll be able to try movements like L-sits, planches, iron crosses, and muscle ups. Wooden rings feel the best and are the highest quality that I know of. Yes, you can buy a $200 TRX set, but why would you if you can just use gymnastic rings. You can use them in conjunction with your dip bar or can take them to the park and hang them off of playground equipment.

- **Dip Bar**: If you can do dips and don't want to invest in gymnastic rings, you'll get a lot of use out of a dip bar. If you're short on space you may want to skip this though because I haven't found a compact dip bar. You're better off just buying a pair of rings.

- **Dip Belt**: Dip belts are great buy. They can be used to make your pull-ups, chin-ups, and dips more challenging. I have one myself and I'm really happy with the purchase.

- **Dumbbells**: This one is pretty obvious, if you're going to workout at home, you'll definitely want some dumbbells for overhead presses, lunges, goblet squats, rows, high pulls, etc. I have two 30lb and two 40lb dumbbells. That's all you'll really need

- **Kettlebells**: Kettlebells have become really popular in the past few years and can be used for kettlebell swings, snatches, Turkish getups, etc. But I don't think they're really necessary. You could technically do those same exercises with dumbbells, so I wouldn't spend money specifically on kettlebells

- **Jump Rope**: Jumping rope is a GREAT way to burn fat. You can jump rope in HIIT (high intensity interval training) format where you jump for 20 seconds, rest for 10, and repeat 8 times. It will build quickness and agility (in addition to burning fat), which is why boxers jump rope so much

- **Medicine Balls**: I wouldn't say that a medicine ball is necessary, but it's useful for medicine ball slams and for throwing (if you have enough space)

- **Bands**: Exercise bands are a good tool to warm up your shoulders. You can do band pull aparts to warm up your shoulders before you do exercises like overhead presses, incline bench presses, and dips. They can also be used across your back to make pushups more challenging. But I wouldn't say that they're absolutely necessary

- **Exercise Bike**: An exercise bike is not necessary, but if you happen to have one at home, you can use it to do bike sprints. In addition to being amazing at burning fat, bike sprints have been proven to help recovery after leg workouts. So if you have one you should definitely use it

- **Treadmill**: Sprints are a FANTASTIC way to burn fat. The problem is that sprints can be dangerous if you don't know the mechanics of running properly, so that's why people recommend sprinting uphill. Well if you don't have a track or a hill nearby, you can set your treadmill at an 8% incline and sprint for 30 seconds followed by 60 seconds of rest (repeat that 5-10 times)

- **Box or Bench**: Having a sturdy workout bench is helpful for doing dumbbell bench presses or incline bench presses. Also having a bench is good for doing box jumps or step ups. If you don't want to buy a bench then you can use a box for box jumps and stepups

So that's all you'll really need. Again, not everything on this list is necessary, but as you progress, you may find it helpful. Also, you can easily find these items at a good price if you shop online.

The ONLY Exercises You Need To Do To Get Ripped at Home

In this section, I breakdown some of the best exercises you can do. Later in this book I'll provide a few sample workout routines, and I'll even show you how to create your own, but here I'm going to list some of my favorite exercises as well as the benefits of doing them.

Bodyweight Strength - Upper Body

- **Pushups**: Pushups are a fantastic exercise for building strength and muscular endurance. They help heal injured shoulders as well (if you've done a lot of bench pressing) and are actually "better" than a bench press because they involve so many different muscle groups. They work your chest, forearms, back, triceps, and abs. The one disadvantage of them is that you can't add weight to them like you can to a bar. But, you can always make them more challenging (I'll explain how below)

- **Elevated Pushups and Pike Pushups**: If regular pushups are too easy for you, you can put your legs up on a bench or on the wall to make them harder. You can also put your legs on a bench or box that is about waist level and do what's called "pike pushups" to make them even harder.

- **Handstand Pushups**: Now handstand pushups are a REAL muscle builder. They are incredibly effective and building powerful shoulders and triceps. They help develop good balance and are a fantastic alternative to overhead presses. The only issue is that there is a somewhat limited range of motion because your head will hit the ground when you go down. The solution to this is to perform them using a pullup bar that is securely on the ground.

- **Plyometric Pushups**: Plyometric pushups have all of the same benefits of regular pushups (and the variations I mentioned above) but they build explosiveness and power. I'll cover plyometrics later in this chapter.
- **Pull-Ups and Chin-Ups**: Pull-ups and chin-ups are awesome exercises because they're compound movements that work multiple muscle groups like your biceps, traps, back, forearms, and abs. You can use multiple hand grips to target your muscles differently.

- **Inverted Rows**: Inverted rows are one of those little known exercises that packs a big punch. They're great at building back and bicep strength and are easier than doing pull-ups. So if you can't do pull-ups, try inverted rows. They're really important to do because people often train their "push" muscles and forget to train their "pull" muscles (i.e. their back) which causes shoulder problems, muscle imbalances, and injuries. So if you aren't doing inverted rows, you should add them to your routine.

- **Dips**: I love dips, they're probably one of my favorite exercises. They're amazing at building your shoulders, triceps, traps, abs, and upper back. When you get more advanced you can use a dip belt to make them more challenging.

Bodyweight Strength Lower Body

- **Pistol Squats/One Legged Squats**: Pistol squats are also known as one-legged squats and they're an incredibly effective test of strength, balance, and coordination. If you can already do them, then you can make them more challenging by holding dumbbells or kettlbells, or by jumping after you've finished performing one rep. They are great at working your glutes, quadriceps, and hamstrings

- Lunges:

- Jump Squats:

Jump squats are very

jump squats

sissy squats

high jumps

lunge jumps

box jumps

Dumbbell Strength Upper Body

db overhead presses

db curls

db high pulls

db incline press

db floor press

db bent over rows

db renegade rows

Dumbbell Strength Lower Body

goblet squats

db front squats

db deadlifts

db bulgarian squats

planks

db getups

db/kb swings

db single leg deadlifts

db good mornings

db step up

CARDIO

mountain climbers

kb swings

jump rope

high knees

high jumps

jump lunges

Variables to Getting the BEST Workout You Can at Home

Yes, the gym is great because of the wide array of equipment, but if you know how to tweak your workouts, you can get an incredibly lean and powerful body.

One of the best ways to get bigger, stronger, and faster is with weights.

But since you probably already know that.

Lifting weights has numerous advantages, regardless of what you use. Dumbbells, barbells, kettlebells, medicine balls, dragging sleds, and of course bodyweight exercises are all useful when trying to get stronger.

I have chosen these exercises very carefully. They give the perfect balance between the following factors:

- **Push vs Pull**: Doing too many pushing movements is bad for your shoulders if you don't balance them with pulling movements. That's why pullups, rows, deadlifts, and face pulls are crucial to main muscular balances and prevent injuries from too much bench pressing

- **Vertical vs Horizontal**: Since we talked about pushing and pulling, it also matters what your position is. For example, the bench press and overhead press are both pushing movements, but one is vertical and one is horizontal. Same with deadlifts and bent over rows; one is done vertically and one is done horizontally. You should use both planes of movement to get a more well-rounded physique

- **Compound vs Isolation Movements:** Doing compound, multi-joint movements is the best way to get the most fat-burning and muscle-building results. You need to do big movements like squats, bench presses, rows, deadlifts, and their variations as well as more isolated movements like curls, calf-raises, and shoulder flyes

- **Volume vs Intensity:** You need to work out very intensely to burn fat and build muscle. You do that in the gym by lifting in reverse pyramid training format. The weight will be heavier, but you're only doing 2 sets and no more than 8 reps per exercise. On your non-gym days, you'll be doing more volume at lighter weight (since you'll be primarily using dumbbells, kettlebells, and bodyweight exercises)

- **Weights vs Bodyweight**: Weights are considered "closed chain" because your body is stationary while the weight moves. Body weight exercises are considered "open chain" because your body moves while the object you're moving against stays stationary (floor, pullup bar, dip bar, etc.) You need to use both free weights and body weight exercises. That way you have BOTH pure strength, and relative strength. Being able to bench press 275 pounds, but not be able to do 5 pullups is not cool. *Plus, body weight exercises like pushups, planks, and back bridges are almost magical for injury prevention and recovery.*

- **Eccentric vs Concentric:** People always ignore their workout tempo but studies have proven that lifting weights explosively and lowering them slowly (about 3-4 seconds) builds fast-twitch muscle fibers, which helps you get stronger, bigger, faster, and more explosive.

So with all that said, let's go into this work that I've been using!

But training *explosive* strength is completely different.

It's one thing to be strong. It's a completely different story to be able to rapidly recruit that strength.

So, what's the best way to build that explosive strength and power?

The #1 way to build explosive strength is through plyometric exercises.

The second best way is to lift your weights and do bodyweight exercises quickly, with _explosive intent._

In this book, I discuss the benefits of plyometric training, as well as some great bodyweight and dumbbell workouts you can use today to burn fat, get lean, and build explosive strength.

Benefits of plyometric training

Plyometric training is one of the best ways to build explosive strength. Below are some reasons to do plyometrics.

Strengthens fast-twitch muscle fibers

The goal of plyometrics is to maximize how fast your muscles contract. Since power is the amount of force exerted in a given amount of time, the quicker your muscles contract, the more powerful you are. This is really helpful in athletics where you have to be able to run, jump, hit, kick, and change directions very quickly. Developing power requires you to train your fast-twitch muscle fibers. Plyometric training works your fast-twitch muscle fibers and teaches your body to "recruit" them faster, resulting in more power.

Increases tendon strength, which means fewer injuries

Strong tendons helps your muscle fibers produce more power. Stronger tendons also means fewer injuries. You make them stronger by placing a controlled stress on them, and providing adequate nutrition and allowing enough time for recovery. When done correctly, plyometrics can help build stronger tendons. But I can't overstate how important it is to warm up thoroughly and rest for a full 2-3 days after each plyometric session.

Otherwise you're doing more harm than good.

Makes your neuromuscular system more efficient

As I mentioned, the stretch-shortening cycle is called into action every time there is a rapid stretching of the muscle spindles. When this happens, a signal is sent from your brain to your muscles via your neuromuscular system. The more efficiently your neuromuscular system can transmit this signal, the faster you can contract and relax your muscles, which in turn increases your speed and power. Plyometric training improves the efficiency of this system.

Improves sports performance

Like I said earlier, plyometric exercises lead to better sports performance. By training your fast-twitch muscle fibers, you can jump higher, punch harder, kick farther, run faster, and decrease the time it takes to exert maximal strength. On top of that, a study in the Journal of Strength & Conditioning Research found that combining squats with plyometric exercises increased hip and thigh power production. That's perfect for sports that require running, jumping, kicking, or twisting.

Plyometric Exercises

Now that we've discussed the importance of doing plyometric exercises and how they build strength, I want to share the 13 best plyometric exercises that you can do. Again, please be sure to warm up thoroughly before doing any of these.

1). Plyometric Pushups

Plyometric pushups, or "clap pushups" are great at building explosive upper body strength. You simply do a pushup and try to push yourself off of the ground.

2). Medicine Ball Throws

Another great upper body plyometric exercise is medicine ball throws. Essentially, you hold a heavy medicine ball and throw it up as fast as you can. It helps to be outdoor when doing this.

3). Depth Jumps

A depth jump is when you drop off of a box or bench and then jump straight up as soon as you hit the ground. It should take less than a fraction of a second. It's a "shock" method that's been proven by Russian researchers to increase vertical jumping ability. It's literally your "secret" weapon if you want to be able to jump higher.

4). Lunge Jumps

With a lunge jump, you start in the lunge position and then explode up into the air. While you're in the air, you switch legs so that you land in the opposite position. For example if you start your lunge with your right foot in front and left one in back, you should land on the ground with your left foot in front and you right foot in back.

5). Rim Jumps

A rim jump is when you stand with both feet flat on the floor and jump straight up, as high as you can. You want to have a target to reach for, like a basketball rim for example, hence the name "rim jumps". To perform this exercise correctly, you need to jump up again as soon as you hit the ground. In that sense, it's similar to depth jumps.

6). Zig Zags

I remember doing zig zags in high school gym class. It's a classic plyometric exercise designed to build speed, quickness, and agility. You simply jump left and right over an imaginary line on the floor.

7) . Sprints

Sprinting is amazing for your health. It helps promote fat loss, builds muscle, and trains your fast-twitch muscle fibers to fire quickly. They're a staple for strength and performance athletes.

8). Single-Leg Deadlifts

The first time I saw these I didn't know what they were. It's when you stand on one leg, hold a dumbbell in your hand, and bend over at the hip. It's a weird looking movement, but good at generating hip power.

9). Pistol Squats

Pistol squats are a classic lower body bodyweight exercise, but we're going to do them with a twist (I know, I know, as if they aren't hard enough on their own). If you can muster up the strength, try to do a jump at the end. It's tough, but will really help increase your lower body explosiveness.

10). Single Leg Calf Raise

To do a single-leg calf raise, you simply stand on a ledge, or low box on the balls of your feet. Then you simply raise up. You can add some weights to your hands if you want, but otherwise you can just hold that position for a few seconds. It obviously works your calf muscles really well.

11). Glute Ham Raise

This is a funny looking exercise, but it really works your hamstrings very well. You may have seen a glute ham raise machine at the gym. If you don't have access to a gym, you simply get on your knees and have someone hold your feet in place. With your torso completely straight, you lower your upper body to the ground until your face is just a few inches from the ground. Feel free to use your arms to keep you from hitting the ground if you aren't strong enough yet.

12). Chair Rockets

"Chair rockets" are a great exercise. You put one foot on a chair or bench with the other one on the ground. Then you explode up, pushing up as if you were climbing a stair. While in the air you want to land on the opposite foot on the chair. As soon as you hit the ground you want to explode back up and do it again. It's almost like a lunge jump, except that it's on a bench or box.

13). Bulgarian Split Squats

Lastly, Bulgarian split squats are another exercise that you can do to build hamstring strength. You stand facing away from a bench and put one foot on the bench (the top of your foot will be on the bench). Then you simply want to squat down, ensuring that all of your weight is on the foot that is on the ground (not the bench). Be sure to keep your back straight the entire time. After that, you repeat the process for your other leg.

14). Pushups

15). Pullups

16). Dips

17). Inverted rows

18). Handstand pushups

19). Elevated pushups

20). Plyometrics can help build explosive power, often without weights. You can mimic this effect with weights by lifting explosively during the concentric part of the movement (the "lifting" part of the lift).

The FASTEST Way to Get Results

If you want to get stronger, you need to **lift weights faster**.

If you want to burn more fat, you need to **lift weights faster**.

If you want to build more muscle, you need to *lift weights faster*.

If you want to build explosive strength, you need to *Lift Weights Faster*.

See where I'm going with this?

Here's a bonus; if you want to double your results, you need to not only lift weights faster, but you should focus on lowering them slowly (**eccentric training**)

But this same technique can be used when working out at home (even with body weight exercises)

In this section, I'm going to reveal why you need to lift weights faster and lower them slower. This technique is so overlooked, so neglected, and so unknown that you'll rarely EVER see anyone use it in the gym.

I'm going show you why you explosive strength training and eccentric lifts are literally the #1 way to skyrocket your strength and muscle gain potential, and how it can help you build a leaner, stronger, more athletic body.

Best of all, it's completely free and you can implement right now.

It can be applied to any type of exercise: Barbells. Kettlebells. Bodyweight exercises. You name it.

So let's get started.

The Usual Suspects

If you want to build more muscle, get stronger, become more athletic, or burn more fat, you have to focus on the tried and true fundamentals. Things like:

- **Progressive overload:** Making sure that you gradually increase the weight or reps over time (link)
- **Proper form:** Make sure that you are lifting correctly and safely (link)
- **Shorter rest intervals:** Resting for less time between sets if you are trying to burn fat (link)
- **"Money" movements:** Make sure you get stronger on your main lifts; the squat, bench press, deadlift, overhead press, dips, pullups, and cleans

Let's say you're a beginner that wants to burn fat and build muscle. Here's what you would do:

- Figure out your macros
- Pick a weight training routine
- Lift weights 3-4 times per week, focusing on compound, multi-joint exercises like squats, bench presses, deadlifts, overhead presses, dips, pullups, and pushups
- You pay attention to your form by watching YouTube videos
- You gradually increase the weight as you get stronger on each movement
- You make sure that you rest enough in between sets (especially if you're strength training)

But eventually, you hit a plateau.

You can't add weight to your lifts for the life of you.

You feel like you've exhausted all of your variables and just can't get any stronger in the gym.

But what if I told you that you could get stronger without lifting heavier weights, or doing more sets and reps?

You'd call me crazy.

What if I told you to start paying attention to workout tempo?

What if I told you to focus on on lifting explosively and lowering the weight slowly (eccentric training), using the exact same weights you're currently lifting with?

Let me explain.

Read below for the reasons to lift weights faster and focus on eccentric training (and how to do both at the same time.

Here are 7 Reasons to Lift Weights Faster

If you're working with a heavy weight (roughly 85% of your 1 rep max), your goal should be to move it as fast as possible during the positive (concentric) part of the motion.

For example, let's say that you're doing a deadlift (you are doing deadlifts aren't you? Here are 13 Reasons You Need to be Deadlifting).

When you pull the bar up from the ground, you want to grip the bar as hard as you can and rip it off the ground, keeping your back, arms, and core straight while keeping the weight in the center of your foot.

You want to do this part quickly, and with purpose.

The positive part of the deadlift (concentric), should be done quickly. That means you want to try to do it as fast as possible, ideally within 1-2 seconds. You literally want to explode the weight off of the ground.

Of course, speed is relative, because if you're using a challenging weight, you won't be able to lift the weight all the way back up in 1-s seconds.

The key here though is *intent*.

That means you should *try* to lift the weight back up as fast as possible. Exploding the weight up recruits your fast-twitch muscle fibers, which are responsible for the greatest size and strength gains.

Still not convinced?

Well, here are 7 reasons to be lifting weights faster.

Reason #1 You Recruit More Muscle Fibers

Researchers discovered a very important law; the faster you lift, the more muscle fibers you recruit.

Lifting weights quickly helps you "recruit" more muscle fibers. That means your body uses more of your muscle fibers. Not only that, but lifting weights fast recruits your fast-twitch muscle fibers; these are the types of muscle fiber that product the greatest size and strength gains.

Muscle fibers (or motor units) are what make your muscles contract. The more muscle fibers your recruit, the bigger, stronger, and faster you become. Oh yeah, and since more muscle burns more calories, you can burn more fat as well.

Here's one way to think about it: your nervous system uses your muscles in an orderly fashion. So if you do low intensity tasks like walking, your body won't use nearly as many muscle fibers as if you were to do a heavy squat. Because you're doing an easy activity, your body uses as little muscle as possible to accomplish that task.

That's why you won't build any muscle by walking or doing any other low intensity activity; your body just isn't challenged enough to call your muscles into action.

Now let's say you started sprinting. Your body will use more muscle fibers because you have to move as fast as possible. You're placing an intense demand on your body, so it responds by activating more muscle. This leads to more muscle growth and greater muscle size. Just look at pictures of sprinters

[insert muscular sprinter picture]

Now there are two main types of muscle fibers; fast-twitch muscle fibers which are responsible for size and strength, and slow-twitch muscle fibers which are mostly responsible for endurance. Lifting weights quickly utilizes the fast-twitch muscle fibers, so if you want to build more muscle and get stronger, lifting faster is the way to go.

Reason #2 You Build Explosive Power

$$Power = \frac{Force \times Distance}{Time}$$

Power is defined as the amount of energy output in a certain amount of time.

Training at a fast rep speed increases the pace at which your muscles can move a given weight. The faster you can move a given weight, the more power you have.

Power is important for overall muscle strength because it helps you accelerate a weight, so increasing power will successfully increase your strength.

When you lift weights explosively, you training your body to not only use more muscle fibers, but you train your body to use them very quickly.

This is very useful for sports like football, martial arts, or baseball where you have to rapidly go from a starting position and explode into a movement.

Box jumps, plyometric pushups, and power cleans are three exercises that come to mind when thinking of power.

When you perform the positive portion of your reps explosively taking less than one second to complete them your fast-twitch muscle fibers are called into action to a greater degree. Fast-twitch muscle fibers produce the greatest muscle force (i.e., strength) and have the highest potential for growth.

Need proof?

University of Alabama researchers recently studied two groups of lifters doing a 29-minute workout. One group performed exercises using a 5-second up phase and a 10-second down phase, the other a more traditional approach of 1 second up and 1 second down. The faster group burned 71 percent more calories and lifted 250 percent more weight than the superslow lifters.

Reason #3 Your Muscle Fibers Work Together Better

So not only do your use more of your muscles and train them to work faster, lifting weights faster trains your muscle fibers to work together, in a more coordinated fashion. Because they are more coordinated, you're stronger.

An example would be someone that wants to increase their vertical jump. Doing box jumps and power cleans would obviously make them stronger and help them jump higher. But doing squats and deadlifts, focusing on exploding up in the concentric part of the lift would also help them because they're using more muscle fibers, training them to react quickly, and coordinating them all to work together.

Not only does this apply to the fibers within a particular muscle group, it also applies to multiple muscle groups. For example, exploding up from the bottom position of a squat trains your body to work your calves, hamstrings, quadriceps, lower back, and core at the same time.

Reason #4 You Can Actually Change Your Muscle Fibers

When you lift weights quickly (with proper form and manageable weight of course), your body adapts by converting your slow-twitch muscle fibers to fast-twitch muscle fibers.

In other words, by applying a specific demand to your body, it adapts and builds stronger, bigger muscles.

Reason #5 You Don't Get Tired as Easily

Another GREAT benefit of lifting weights fast is that you get as tired. Rather than feeling dead tired (like if you just ran a long distance) you feel energized and revved up.

Don't get me wrong, I'm tired after I deadlift, or squat, or bench press, or overhead press because I'm lifting at 85% to 90% of my 1 rep max.

BUT, as long as you aren't grinding your reps (that means it's too heavy, or you're doing too many reps) you'll feel good lifting faster

So to recap, you want to lift weights fast during the positive portion of the exercise. It doesn't need to be done in 1 second, but that should be your goal. Doing this activate more muscle, train your body to fire more quickly, and teach your body to coordinate not only the muscle fibers, but the major muscle groups as well. Chad Waterbury wrote a great article on T-Nation about this same topic.

https://www.t-nation.com/training/3-reasons-to-lift-explosively

6 Reasons to Lower the Weights Slowly (Eccentric Training)

Now let's talk about the reasons to focus on eccentric training.

Eccentric training is when you purposely slow down the negative phase (eccentric phase) of a lift. So rather than speeding through a rep on the bench press, you purposely, slowly lower the bar. This should take you 3-4 seconds.

Now, lots of guys think that they should do their entire lift slowly, and based on what I've said earlier, you might think that you should do the entire part of the lift quickly, but that's not the case. The problem with lifting too quickly is that you end up relying on momentum, which minimizes tension and overload on the muscles. Plus you run the risk of getting hurt.

So lifting weights slowly reduces momentum and activates your target muscles more. It also forces you to focus on proper form and use a manageable weight. It also allows you to focus on the mind-muscle connection, your breathing, etc.

Lifting weights slowly has a lot of benefits.

The key is to do the negative part of the movement slowly. Below are 6 reasons to slow down the eccentric (negative) part of the movement:

Reason #1 New Muscle Growth

Eccentric training is the deliberate deceleration of weight, which naturally increases the intensity of the exercise. It also gives a different stimulus to the muscle group because of the longer "time under tension". This causes the target muscle to adapt, which leads to bigger, stronger muscles.

Reason #2 Higher Anabolic Hormonal Output

The human body is amazing.

Anytime it's introduced to an external stimulus or stress, it's natural response is to release high amounts of anabolic hormones.

You know, like the kinds that bodybuilders inject to get bigger and stronger.

But there's only one exception; your body produces them naturally.

Hormones like testosterone, human growth hormone (HGH), and insulin-like growth factor (IGF-1).

By lowering a heavy set of weights slowly, you tell your neuro-endocrine system to flood your system with these hormones, causing your body to burn body fat, build muscle, increase bone density, and turbo-charge sex drive.

Reason #3 Increased Metabolism

Eccentric training is more intense. So your muscles have no choice but to adapt and grow. A side affect of muscle growth is increased metabolism.

Bye-bye fat. Hello muscle.

Let me say it clearly; eccentric training, especially paired with the right diet will help scorch body fat while simultaneously preserving muscle by adding more intensity to your training, WITHOUT adding more weight, frequency, or volume to your lifting regimen.

Reason #4 Increased Muscular Endurance

Now this isn't rocket science, so I'm not going to explain it in detail.

But when you lower the weight slowly, your muscles develop more oxidative capacity.

That basically means you can burn through your current endurance threshold.

Simply put, you can lift more weight for longer.

Reason #5 Muscle Preservation During Dieting

If you're dieting you're going to lose fat.

But you'll also lose stored glycogen, water, and yes, muscle.

Sad but true… unless you use steroids (well, maybe even if you use steroids)

Bottom line: limiting calories will most likely cause you to lose muscle and strength.

However, studies have shown that engaging in highly intense eccentric loading exercise, anabolic hormones such as testosterone, HGH and IGF-1 help preserve muscle mass, even during caloric restriction.

So here's the good news: if you're dieting you probably will lose muscle and strength, but eccentric training helps preserve your gains.

So lower those weights slowly.

Reason #6 Enhanced Overall Athletic Performance

Whether you're a professional athlete or an avid gym goer, trainees see incredible changes in their overall strength, speed, explosiveness and power when they focus on lowering the weight in a slow, controlled manner.

By focusing on lowering weights slowly, you'll notice an improvement in your vertical reach, punching power, throws, or any other athletic movement .

Putting It All Together

So I'm saying to lift the weights faster, which means you want to *try* to lift the weight within 1 to 2 seconds (intent is the key)

And I'm also saying that you want to lower the weight slowly, within about 3-4 seconds.

If you can't do either, the weight is probably too heavy.

If the weight's too heavy you'll probably end up using poor form.

If you use poor form, you'll probably end up hurting yourself.

[insert pic of poor form, or someone hurting themselves]

And hurting yourself is the fastest way to get weak and fat.

So you want to use a weight that you can manage (85% of your 1 repetition max) and do the concentric movement fast and the eccentric movement slow.

Again, you can do this with squats, presses, and deadlifts, but you can also do it with pushups, pullups, and dips.

Basically, this is relevant to any kind of resistance exercise.

Two Simple Home Workouts You Can Use Today

I like to lift weights these days, but I'm in love with bodyweight exercises. Pushups, pullups, burpees, jump squats, mountain climbers, and my all time favorite; dips. I can't get enough of them.

I know Todd has a TON of great workouts, so I wanted to share the one that I personally do. If you're just getting started, don't worry because we're going to take it slow in the beginning. But over time we'll add more repetitions. You'll notice yourself getting stronger and leaner in the process.

Each week, you want to add 3-5 more reps and 1 more set. There are no hard and fast rules here. The point is to do a little bit more each week than you did the previous week.

PURE BODYWEIGHT WORKOUT:

- Monday: 10 pushups followed by 10 burpees followed by 5 pullups. Rest one minute and repeat 2 more times (the following week you can do 15 pushups, 15 burpees, and 6 pullups or the you can do 4 total rounds with the same number of repetitions, and so forth each week)

- Tuesday: 5 burpees followed by 5 split squats followed by 5 mountain climbers, followed by 5 high knees. Rest one minute and repeat 2 more times (again, the next week you can add more repetitions or more

- Wednesday: 10 pushups followed by 10 burpees followed by 5 pullups. Rest one minute and repeat 2 more times (the following week you can do 15 pushups, 15 burpees, and 6 pullups or the you can do 4 total rounds with the same number of repetitions, and so forth each week)

- Thursday: 5 burpees followed by 5 split squats followed by 5 mountain climbers, followed by 5 high knees. Rest one minute and repeat 2 more times (again, the next week you can add more repetitions or more

- Friday: 10 pushups followed by 10 burpees followed by 5 pullups. Rest one minute and repeat 2 more times (the following week you can do 15 pushups, 15 burpees, and 6 pullups or the you can do 4 total rounds with the same number of repetitions, and so forth each week)

As you get stronger, add more reps, or even another exercise like dips, or wall pushups, or pistol squats on Monday, Wednesday, and Friday or to cut your rest time from 1 minute to 30 seconds. The key is to progressively make the workouts harder as you get stronger.

This workout is so easy that it can be done in less than 25 minutes. If you have kids (like me), you can do this with them at the park, or at home. You're going to have to figure out how to keep them from jumping on your back when doing pushups though! (sorry, no suggestions for you there)

The benefit of doing this workout is that you naturally combine resistance training with high intensity cardio; allowing you to build muscle and burn fat.

A Sample Week of Workouts (*You Can Do This Now*)

Welcome to day 2 of my course. I wanted to give you something really actionable that you can use right now.
So here's a workout you can do right now. You want to do it for 3 weeks straight. When you do it, keep this in mind:

- BE SURE TO WARM UP TO PREVENT INJURY: some pushups, squats, and pullups will do the trick
- Choose weights that you can comfortably manage, but that still challenge you
- Every week, try to increase the amount of weight by 5 lbs

- Do all 3 exercises immediately after each other and take 1 minute rest when you're done. This will trigger the EPOC effect where you burn calories after your workout because the intensity is so high
- Be sure to eat protein 20 minutes afterwards: edamame, greek yogurt, tuna, etc.

Within 15 days, you WILL see and feel a noticeable change in your physique. And you'll be motivated to eat right and keep up with the program.

Monday: **(do each set 4-5 times w/ 1 minute rest between sets)**
Barbell Squats x 8 (135 lbs)
Dumbbell Press Ups x 8 (45 lbs per dumbbell)
Burpees x 8

Wednesday: **(do each set 4-5 times w/ 1 minute rest between sets)**
One Arm Dumbbell Power Snatch x 8 (45 lbs per dumbbell)
One Arm Dumbbell Push Jerk x8 (45 lbs per dumbbell)
Box Jumps (or Squat Jumps) x 8

Friday: **(do each set 4-5 times w/ 1 minute rest between sets)**
Romanian Deadlifts x 6 (45 lbs per dumbbell)
Dumbbell High Pulls x 6 (45 lbs per dumbbell)
Lunges w/ Alternating Dumbbell Presses x 6 (45 lbs per dumbbell)
Dumbbell Hang Clean and Squat x 6 (45 lbs per dumbbell)

Printed in Poland
by Amazon Fulfillment
Poland Sp. z o.o., Wrocław

35443763R00027